Made in United States
North Haven, CT
26 October 2021

10590795R00068